THE FUNDAMENTALS OF MENTAL HEALTH RECOVERY

Raheem Cox

ISBN: 979-8-218-42043-7

A mental cage is the worst cage. Twenty-first-century America is becoming more and more fast-paced. Don't get left behind.

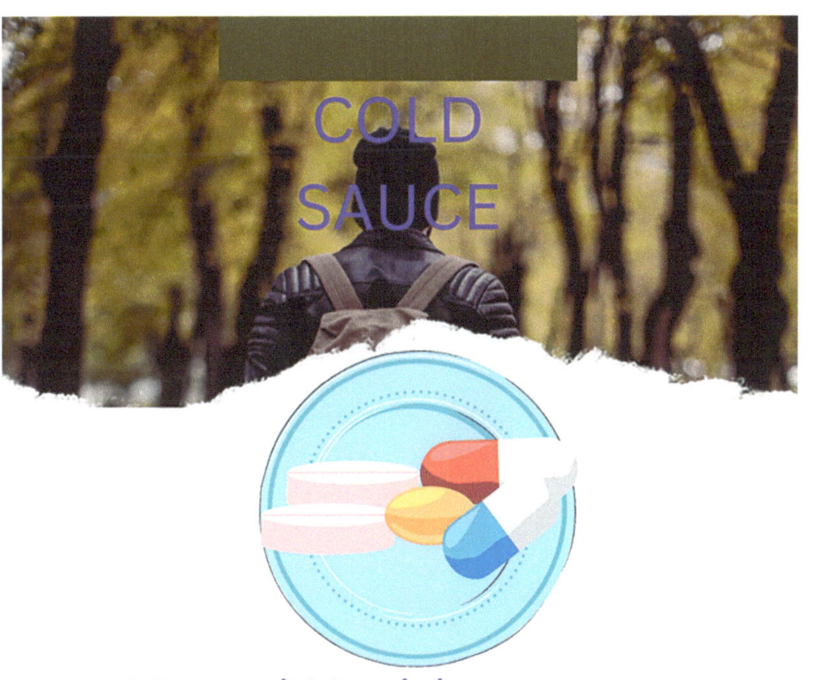
COLD
SAUCE
Mental Health awarenss
podcast

Contents

INTRODUCTION

We all need to learn the fundamentals of having better mental health. The contents of this book, *The Fundamentals of Mental Health Recovery*, are derived from one of the best mental health podcasts out. This book is an offshoot of a more extensive book called *From Mentally Ill to Mentally Rich*, which I recommend you also read. This is short in comparison but very effective for treating mental illness. This country has many advantages over others. However, the hardships within trigger many mental health issues. When reading this book, listen to the little things I quote and state. In each episode that I cast biweekly via www.rootforcepublications.com, I made sure to give my full effort and to be highly mindful, responsible, and professional. The episodes are cast by someone that has endured the many sides of mental illness. What I did was I took my history of mental health problems and documented it into a podcast. *The Fundamentals of Mental Health Recovery* discusses prime teachings that I believe are universal to all with mental health problems for their treatment and recovery. Everyone who has had the chance to listen to my podcast *Cold Sauce* mentioned that the contents within and how it all was uniquely put together were very beneficial to their mental health. I took the timeline of mental health history in the United States, knowing that most mental health consultants in this country are not effective enough and need the assistance and viewpoints of someone with a history of mental health issues. This book is the outcome.

COPING WITH MENTAL ILLNESS

Instructing how to cope with mental illness is highly difficult. You should know this first off: When someone is trying to treat your mental health problems, it could be a strain because a normal citizen can't relate to where you're coming from. Now I know you expect to see a psychiatrist or someone with a degree or a doctorate for awareness. But that person is also almost in the same position as a normal person. You are the best person to address your problem at hand. Oftentimes, the best way to deal with your problems is to gain awareness. Many start off wrong, just sitting around with the same mental drawback for years at a time and not trying to gain any knowledge or understanding of their problem. And this can dampen, block, or overindulge their mind to the point they are distraught.

As for me, I've been dealing with mental health problems for many years. I've been in and out the psych ward until I realized I do have a mental illness. First off is admitting it, stating that you do have a mental illness. But stating that you do have that problem can make you seem weak. You should know that just because you have a mental illness doesn't mean that you're weak. It could mean that you're talented in other areas that require a little bit more endurance for the time being. The stigma behind mental illness is what could dampen down people's spirits the most. Its stigma can largely affect how other people look at you. Family and friends can impact your mind heavily. Instilling confidence within the mental health community is key.

I broadcast *Cold Sauce* because of the fact that I'm experiencing mental health issues and can advise a little bit better than a doctor or a therapist with your mental health problems. I feel that I'm the best fit to address mental health problems as I'm someone that has these problems himself. Coping with these problems comes down the line. From my experience, for 70–90 percent of people that have or have had mental illness, the first stage is addressing that they have it but not really coping with it. There are some out there that from the start can diagnose their problem, gain awareness, and treat it all in one. That start is a shock. You might not be able to cope with it at first. Actually, having mental health problems could mean that the Lord probably has something in store for you that requires you to pack a large load for the time being.

Life is a test. Once you notice that, you can stand up to the upheaval. Every case is different. There's bipolar disorder, schizophrenia, and depression. And all of these are diagnosed differently depending on a particular patient. A lot of medical staff are intelligent, but they're looking only at facts, which can distill their mind. You're looking at this person that's highly intelligent, and the information they're telling you can deter your mind. You're just looking at this person and thinking, "I'll never be able to reach their level, so why should I bother?" So to cope with mental illness, the first thing to do is to gain awareness and confidence. I've been in and out of psych wards plenty of times. The best way to cope with mental illness is to know that there is assistance out here to help you gain awareness. Oftentimes, your mental illness is still quite serious because you're in a setting that you have no control over.

That's where the problem comes in. For someone that's mentally ill, the best thing to do is to reach out to someone in your community. It's essentially up to you to pinpoint your problem. Remember the word "pinpoint." You have to pinpoint your problem first to get over with it. If you are tuning in to this episode of *Cold Sauce*, you should first know that the field of psychiatric treatment is diverse. There are new illnesses popping up every day. Mental illness is a very widespread issue. Let me give you a coping mechanism that can better suit you to know more about your illness. I'm sure many of you out there have internet access. Go to Google and type in a keyword, and you will find information about your mental illness. Reading is also very fundamental.

After publishing my first book, *Critical Standpoint*, I published another called *See the Box before It Seats You*. It talks about how illiteracy levels are directly linked to mental illness. Know this: the best things in life are free. Reach out and attach yourself to things that people cannot take away from you. I'm sure many of you out there have documentation. Reading anything is very beneficial. Exercise is also very good. First, for someone with mental illness, having no coping mechanism could make life highly difficult because the pace of life in America is very fast. Normal citizens don't have time to slow down what they're doing. You have to have it in you to overcome your problem. Normal people don't have time to sit down and cater to your issue. I haven't had too many mental setbacks in the past years. I took everything one step at a time. I came to the conclusion that I did have a problem, which I, at first, didn't want to admit. My first step was admitting that I did have that problem. It was a stepping stone to getting better. After admitting that, I started reading and then reaching out to the mental health community in my city. New York City has a lounge where people can communicate. If you have internet, check around to see what's available to you. Like I said, every case is different. First, know there is a way to get over it. It's mainly pinpointing your problem. Maybe your mental illness is normal. Maybe it's not that uncommon. Maybe there's something unique that you're doing that requires a little bit more mental strain. Mental illness is not always uncommon. Climate, temperature, and the environment are very important to the mental health community. You currently might feel a bit drawn back, but if you examine seasonal factors, you would have been in that mental state anyway. This is one of the most important things I could have stated in this podcast episode. Sometimes, even if the trigger to your mental problems isn't current, you would have been in that state anyway. Your mental problems could have been something normal. Why do you think the greats of the world (scientists, athletes, and politicians) have mental problems? First, you have to look at how someone of that stature could have achieved what they had despite having difficulty functioning. Another thing that I want to point out is you have to be a better listener. Being a good observer and listener is vital to your status. It can open up a way to see your deficit down the line. It's very important to find a hobby that you like as this can boost your confidence.

THE ECONOMY AND MENTAL HEALTH

First off, what is mental health? Mental health is a person's condition involving their psychological and emotional well-being. Then there's the economy, which is the wealth or resources of a country or region. What I want to do in this particular episode is show the relationship between a nation's current economy and a citizen's mental health status, which are interrelated. Many mentally ill people are so dampened down and stressed by life that they can't see how the economy is the primary factor that is negating or worsening their mental health status. I've had these problems within the mental health community for over a decade now. Why did I choose to document this particular episode? It's because while I was a young man in psychiatric hospitals and outpatient treatment programs, I was so dampened down by life, and those around me had similar problems.

The economy can affect your mental health status. I wanted to show that oftentimes, the economy and the governance within your state or region are the primary factors that negate or worsen your mental health. What I want to point out is that these elected US officials are, in large part, no different from someone with a mental health issue. Yes, they could be a little bit more educated and able to adapt to being a member of a board or a committee. In my earlier years, I was so broken that I couldn't see the relationship between the economy and my mental health status. A lot of times, people with mental health problems don't even assess their treatment. Oftentimes, their treatment can be a little bit better. A lot of times, psychiatrists tell you the same thing over and over, like taking your pills.

Sometimes someone like me that has mental problems can break down the factors that are setting them back. Let's go back to elected officials: Their daily lifestyle is not that different from yours. They drink and party. These are the same people that have passed guidelines and laws that set the general standards in your community. These are the same people that dictate what's right and wrong or just how footed you are as a person or citizen in your community. Don't just sit back and let your government overpower you with their educational status, as if you can't gain awareness or insight. I'm sure you have mental problems. But I'm also sure you can read, listen, and observe. Work on things that others can't take away from you. Don't let the American economy deprive you of your share of happiness.

I know how it is with someone with mental health problems: their mind is so shelled or fractured to the point where the economy is out of reach. The economy and how it's run are things that are far out of reach for someone with mental problems. Read or watch the news. You don't have to read for hours a day. Awareness is key. The peak or increase in one area leads to a low in another area. Only the stereotypes of mental health are portrayed on American media. A lot of times, the government forms the current mindset that you're in. The purpose of this episode was to show this. Channels like MTV, BET, and VH1 show stereotypes like doing drugs in school, having sex at an early age, ridiculing certain groups of people, and that it's cool to be uneducated. Oftentimes, these stereotypes in media have a big impact on your mental status. A lot of times, they are what cause your mental health issues in the first place. You have to pinpoint the cause of your mental problems.

Ninety percent of the time, the only way you can break out of your mental problems is by first noticing it. Mood swings are due to your normal mental status being thrown out of whack. The economy, in general, can paint an image that can throw you off your equilibrium. Now within the mental health community, "equilibrium" is a very important term. The maintenance of a person and the maintenance of an economy are very similar. In the maintenance of a person, you're dealing with hygiene, eating right, and clothing. Congress is a system of checks and balances. They have board meetings, where they discuss matters and weigh odds and ends. They converse. They communicate. What I want to point out is don't let these people in Congress overpower you and tell you what's sanctionable and what's not sanctionable.

Right now, think about the last hospital you were in or the last treatment you had. Why do you think they said the same things, mentioned the same terms, or made the same suggestions? Why was their evaluation of you very similar to or shared the same guidelines within their facilities? The same policies that employees that work in these facilities need to follow are very similar too, and their willingness to help you is very similar. That's because everything starts with Congress, the economy included. Oftentimes, you're so out of whack mentally that you can't see the daily lives of elected officials are very similar to that of a normal person. Sometimes they do wrongful things. I'm sure you heard in the papers about elected officials getting caught. At first, mental problems at be avoided. If I could turn back time, I would listen to a podcast like this to educate myself on the legislative body that dictates how the economy is run as well as mental health concerns. When you gain awareness, you're doing a lot more for yourself than you think you are. When I was around sixteen or seventeen, I wasn't aware yet how the government was run—that is, until my late twenties. As I mentioned in the last episode, I was on the honor roll in high school, but I didn't understand how the economy and a person's lifestyle were so interrelated.

I speak to a lot of peers within the mental health community. At some point in a person's life, you need to gain awareness. You don't need to be a judge or a state assemblyman or a city councilman. But you need to gain awareness on how your government is run. The mental health community is very similar to paying off debts and liabilities. A country's productiveness plus its citizens' dissatisfaction with their country equals the overall general happiness of a country. It's similar to a business balance sheet. Access plus liabilities equals owner's equity. The mental health community is composed of drug addicts, members of families that are shied away from, and employees trying to keep up with certain standards that are hard to keep up with. I hope I illustrated the correlation between the economy and mental health as clear as possible.

LIVING VAGUE TURNS INTO A PLAGUE

Vagueness which is lacking expression of. Those living under that detailed definition for a long period of time that is the beginning stages of what caused their mental illness. This is connected not only to the mental health community but also to people with normal mental health. A lot of times, you don't have the necessities within your place of residence to promote your own progress. As a man or woman, you were meant to fill the gap. You were meant to have well-being. You were meant to achieve things. Some people spend their time doing unrealistic things that have no value to it. Like the saying goes, idle hands are the devil's workshop, and it comes back to hurt you in the long run. That's the case for a lot of people with mental illness. What I notice is that 90 percent of the time, the lack of exhibiting ambition to the American youth is the prime factor that caused their mental illness. Right now, post-corona kids are flunking out of schools in great masses. The public school system is really not getting it done anymore. There aren't many places to exhibit your talents in the American infrastructure.

And a lot of times, that vagueness turns into a plague. Mental illness spreads. It's more common knowledge than anything. Someone with a lack of will or positivity turns to hurt the entire neighborhood, especially if this person is viewed as a role model. A scientific observation that relates very heavily to this episode is our brains are wired to be highly efficient, working at a high level. The human body is very complex. You were made to fill the gap and to be doing something purposeful. The way the human body and brain work is like a miracle. You're dealing with many components of the body that all work together, and when there's a lack in a portion of it, the entire body shuts down. For instance, if you were to take out a chip or component in a computer, radio, or television, it would prevent that equipment from functioning. Your brain is wired to operate at a highly efficient level, so when you're living vague, you're stopping the body from functioning properly. How bipolar disorder leads to schizophrenia or schizophrenia to depression is a tight correlation. You're going to overwork yourself naturally. Sometimes doubt is a good thing. Why does living vague turn into a plague? You weren't born with a highly efficient brain and body just to be living with little to no ambition. Just know when you live every day improperly, it's only a matter of time before your body suffers. You have to understand the makeup of the body. In the present day, living vague is something you almost can't avoid, especially in urban communities.

Mental illness, in a large sense, is like a clogged drain in the mind over a long period of time. You are your own worst enemy. It's up to you what to do with your personal time. If you don't know too much about nature, it naturally balances things out. You can't just say, "There's a lack of opportunity, so I'm not going to promote my own progress." You have to adjust in some other way in any part of the world on a daily basis. Your ambition, for the most part, is something you have control over. I'm sure you have a 99¢ store, library, or park where you can go to in the community so you can express yourself. In just about every neighborhood, there's something that you can take home from stores to help you see things a little bit clearer and more coherently.

DRUG ADDICTION AND MENTAL HEALTH

Being mentally ill is oftentimes caused by marijuana and alcohol abuse. For this particular episode, I'm not going to discuss hard drugs like cocaine and crack cocaine because they're almost certain to cause the deterioration of mental health. Most people started drug use early on. A lot of people started experimenting with drugs for the first time in high school. Drugs are very difficult to avoid because American culture, in large part, is exposed to much drug use, especially in how the media portrays it. It's funny how drug use can seem like a good thing in the beginning, but it becomes a problem when it turns into drug abuse that leads to mental illness. You don't want to be dependent on drugs to bring happiness in life.

It turns into a problem when you try to use drugs to gain happiness. If you use marijuana or alcohol and are able to control it, so be it. I was heavily affected by drug use in my teenage years, and it played a large role in my mental health. The majority of the time I was sent to psychiatric hospitals was because I couldn't control my drug addiction. People use drugs for many different reasons. Sadly, it's almost unavoidable because of how US legislature deals with the matter. You go from the school system to a later day in living and rise up the school system. If you're fortunate enough to go to college or to find employment, it's important to do something useful with your time. People utilize their time differently. People from middle-income to low-income neighborhoods go from point A to point B to point C, and it's very hard for these people to avoid drug abuse. There aren't many ways for the less fortunate to express themselves, and a lot of the time, this can lead to a mental illness. Not everyone has the discipline to pick up a drug that alleviates and soothes your mind and is very beneficial to your life. In current-day America, 38 percent of the 20 million adults with substance abuse problems have been diagnosed with some sort of mental illness, which is a good portion showing that it's common. I'm not speaking about drugs like marijuana and alcohol as I believe these would not be issued if the authorities didn't feel like they could be used under fair and safe standards. You shouldn't have any problem with cigarettes either. Drug abuse is the problem. Oftentimes, psychiatric medicine doesn't have a favorable reaction to someone that's mentally ill.

Recovering fully from drug addiction, where the individual could regain some form of balance in their life, could take months or even years. I hate to knock drugs too heavily because they're often all the mentally ill have to block mental agony. I know what it feels like to have voices in your head—like the world is wreaking havoc on your life. Like I mentioned earlier, there aren't many ways to express yourself when you come from a low- or middle-income household. Other than school and sports, America is set up so that drug usage is the norm, making it very hard to avoid. The history of drug use goes back thousands of years. The drug trade, in general, is something that probably won't go away in your lifetime. Not to think too much like a square, if you're responsible, it's not a problem. There are two types of people: (1) someone that uses drugs heavily and never has any mental dysfunction and (2) someone that uses the same drug heavily but can't function. So I asked myself, "Where does the difference come in?" Oftentimes, the answer depends on one's mentality or how healthy or able a person is to balance the effects of the drug. Once, I received advice from someone. He said, "You're not crazy. Your thoughts are just mixed up. A lot of people have some form of mental illness. They're normal people. It's just their mentality is not strong enough yet. A lot of times, the task at hand doesn't fit well into their lifestyle." Sometimes your mentality is not strong enough to balance the effects of the drug. Abusing drugs while mentally ill oftentimes puts a blindfold over you where you can't see how you're treating yourself and others.

As you're listening to this episode right now, you're probably thinking, "He answered my problems in a way but didn't touch on certain matters." That's because the relationship between drug addiction and mental health is a very broad topic. If you find yourself abusing drugs and still haven't found an alternative route, especially if you are still an adolescent or juvenile, you have to change your plans. Certain members of society make good use of their time to balance the effects of drug use. Drugs can do some good for people that are mentally ill, so I'm not going to sit here and downplay their effects because oftentimes they're all you have. Just be responsible. Or seek therapy if you can or reach out to someone that you can speak to about your problems.

READ, LISTEN, AND OBSERVE

Being vague-minded doesn't get you anywhere, and being an average joe doesn't get you anywhere either. Regarding those that rose in rank in society or hold high-ranking jobs, you will probably find that they share this one thing in common: they made great efforts to enlighten themselves. You get nothing from being dull-minded and simple. This is why reading, listening, and observing are so important. Many average Americans don't see the importance of being good to one another. A lot of them are very foul-tempered. It is hard to subsist in this country. Existence alone can sometimes be a strain. I just read in an article that being a good employee or person stems mostly from preparing yourself for the agenda ahead. And reading, listening, and observing help in this. It's what separates the conscious from the unconscious. It's one of the best skills to master. Take advantage it's free. For those that are afflicted by bipolar disorder, schizophrenia, and mood swings, I'm not trying to tell you how to spend your time. But being mindful is a trait that can help you in many other areas.

The unique ways that people read, listen, and observe make the world go round. When some people read, they skim. They read a couple of words in a paragraph and skip to the next, whereas others read thoroughly. Some people listen to everything someone is saying, while some are selective listeners. When some people observe, they're just looking at things that are interesting to them, while others are able to bring out the beauty of whatever it is they're observing. How the greats of this world viewed the world was very distinct. Most of them read documents and enlightened themselves in a manner that significantly impacted them. Most of them looked at particular things under magnifying lens, and this made them who they are. I know it's hard to do that when you can't see the dignity in life. When life is too hard, you don't want to read. It may seem odd or may seem unclear, but reading, listening, and observing are probably the best ways to recover from mental illness. Why? Right now, just think back to the times you were receiving psychiatric treatment, and they handed out fact sheets on your particular mental illness for the first time. The details you read actually helped you in more ways than you perceive. When you picked up documents in your psychiatric classes and were told what your mental illness was, they gave you something similar to an initial vaccine. Reading gives you a sense of awareness that will nurture your mind, and enlightening yourself gives you the intelligence to be able to give someone feedback that could make you seem like a more reasonable person.

When grouped together, reading, listening, and observing are very purposeful when you're doing all three the right way. For me personally, it significantly boosts my self-esteem. A decade or so ago, it came to a point when I told myself I had to improve my viewpoints. After reading, I stepped it up to listening. Then I stepped it up to observing. This made the professional writer that I am today. What's not spoken about is if you do all three the right way prior and up until recovering from your mental illness, you will be five to ten times stronger than you once were. Oftentimes, people that had it the hard way are a lot more mindful, but they're just not in the position to say it. Just about nothing can be done with a simple theory of looking at things. It is important to fill each of your days with something purposeful. It's about playing a sport and using the right skill and technique. Reading, listening, and observing are all rudimentary activities that lead to enlightenment. This is why I documented this particular episode.

MOOD SWINGS ARE NORMAL

Those with mental health problems, on average, are antagonized by mood swings on a daily basis. It is almost impossible for the average person to go without them. Many lack understanding of their imbalance: imbalance of traits and characteristics and things that shape emotions. They don't realize mood swings are actually normal. When you're so stigmatized by people judging your character from the outside, it makes you criticize yourself down to the smallest detail. Mentally ill people are viewed as having an abnormal character. Let's look at one thing that causes mood swings: loss of energy. This is something anyone can fall victim to because a lot of people are not financially stable enough to feed themselves properly or provide themselves the proper necessities to balance out the imbalance of mood swings.

Let's take a look at another one: hopelessness. Many employees come by hopelessness during their time working. This can include lacking the motivation to handle tasks. Sometimes a task is overwhelming, or an employer is placing too much burden on an employee. So hopelessness is fairly normal.

Let's look at another one: difficulty concentrating. One can have difficulty concentrating when a lighting fixture is not properly put in place, and the lighting overhead can lower your concentration levels and shift your consciousness, which can throw off your mental balance. It can come from a window being opened too wide that you have no control over closing or shutting, and the resulting cold breeze can cause an irritation in your mental status.

I will discuss another one: restlessness. It could come from anything: not eating the right diet, not knowing what your particular diet is, too much pressure at work, too packed a work schedule to be able to wake up the next day.

What I found similar among people with mental health problems is that their mental, spiritual, and physical states have many lacks. You have to start getting rid of some of the problems you encounter on a daily basis. A lot of people with mental health problems don't understand the following: They have to learn to eat right. They have to learn to exercise right. They have to learn to wear proper clothing. Sometimes you're living too vague, and you don't have the mental capacity to say, "If I'm doing nothing all day, I'm breaking down my mind." A lot of people with mental problems don't interact the right way with other people. They throw themselves out there. They say idle hands are the devil's workshop. A lot of people with mental health problems break themselves down by living in an abnormal state. From experience, about 80–90 percent of people with mental health problems have symptoms that can't be turned around.

Just speaking on the last year in general, I focused mainly on taking a shower, brushing my teeth, and using mouthwash. But I found out that when I focused too heavily on one part, I could never remember to do the other parts consistently. For instance, hygiene includes all the things that keep your mental status, behavior, and character at an equilibrium.

And the moral of this episode is it's hard to keep up with all of them, so mood swings are normal. Whether you're at an outdoor or indoor setting, your body is triggered by many things around you: the climate, the roughness of the floor you're standing on, the objects around you, how the air around you smells.

A lot of times, people with mood swing disorders look at themselves as abnormal. The fact is a lot of mood swings are caused by things that take the ability to balance a lot of factors. More mood swings can ridicule you to the point where you're fed up. Take it one step at a time. Correct things around you. If you can see the normality of mood swings, you will be able to diagnose your problem a lot faster.

EPISODE 7

HONOR THY MORNING

Morning has much value to someone that is mentally ill that wants to recover. I'm sure you heard when you were young that morning is a very symbolic time of day. Those that are successful in this world mastered their daily routine early on. Cleanliness is next to godliness—honoring thy morning almost has the same correlation. I've been in many different stages. If I had just taken things one step at a time and valued the small steps instead of trying to recover overnight, I probably would have recovered a lot faster. If I could take back time, I would try to understand honoring my morning. Now that I'm at the age of thirty-five, I've realized that what helped me the most in my recovery process was mainly honoring my morning. I found the value of my morning. That's what helped me break out significantly. Honoring thy morning is not as simple as I'm explaining right now.

Among the worst things in this world include not being able to go bed at night and not waking up to a good morning. During my mental trauma, it would take me two to three hours to go to sleep. It's also preparing for honoring your morning. What really is "honoring your morning"? When first awakening, you see your past, present, and a more vivid glimpse into your future. So the morning is like an indefinite way to rebalance yourself. If you understand the structure of a mechanism, you understand that everything starts from down low. Your senses are most keen upon just waking up. That goes for just about anybody. If you observe a little bit more and are a little bit more astute to living before going to bed, you will have a much more pleasant time dealing with living. Your morning is like an indefinite resolution to narrow down your body's deterioration.

I mentioned in my earliest segment the importance of pinpointing your problem. The morning is like a breaking point to pinpoint your problem. It's almost like a free gift for you to adopt. I couldn't break out of my mental illness until I corrected my mistakes from morning to night. If your morning doesn't complement you in some way, you're probably doing something wrong. This means you have to sacrifice something. For many people with a mental illness and within the mental health community, it's very common to reason with their mental illness. The way US legislature is handed down, they want you to be lazy. They want you to have to feed off their means of living to subsist. Most successful people are successful because they have exhibited taking part in in the morning.

KNOW YOUR TRIGGERS IN AND OUT

Triggers for both the mentally ill and just about any citizen are common. These triggers could be a sight, a sound, a smell, a physical sensation, a time of day, or a season. If you don't know your triggers, there's a saying that goes "Insanity is doing the same thing over and over and expecting different results." So if you are living under a mental lack or living a lifestyle that is too fast and haven't had the time to sit still and find the humbleness inside you, you have to pinpoint your triggers. You should know them in and out. Knowing your triggers in and out is key to recovering from mental illness. It is common to not notice your triggers until you get older or reach a certain level of mental illness. Some people can spot them early and never have mental illness ever again. A lot of people can't spot their mental triggers early on because they've had these triggers since childhood. Without drug use in my teens, I probably would've been deprived of certain recreation of fair standards. In lower-class communities we were not offered that much. Programs and assistance to help lower-class citizens to reach a higher level of enlightenment were absent. So it's normal to have two or three triggers that commonly throw them off. Know your rights and educate yourself so the next generation can avoid the obstacles you faced. Knowing your triggers in and out is an important aspect of enlightenment in general.

It is a process that may require you to take away the fun out of life. Knowing your triggers in and out also means understanding your life, your neighborhood, your diet, and your hygiene. Know these things first. This way, you could come to a realization of self, your understanding is better, and you can cope with the mental determent of your brain. Knowing your triggers in and out is a very deep aspect of enlightenment. There's always going to be things in your environment that trigger you off from a normal mental health status. It could be lack of financial aid. It could be a family member. It could be a boss at work that is hard to deal with. Or you haven't found out how to maintain proper hygiene.

Why I'm so successful with five books under my belt right now is because I took the time to build a strong core value and embraced things around me that made me resilient to my surroundings. A portion of my mental illness may never fade away. But for the most part, I am happy. I would've never been as successful as I am today if I didn't take the time to instill a core value. If you know your triggers in and out, your day will be running very smoothly. Knowing your triggers in and out involves knowing them not only in one setting but in different settings as well. When you step out the house, how do you feel? You have to understand your body in and out. What triggers you when you get in the car? What triggers you when you are face-to-face with a particular person? What is it about this scenario? You have to know your body in and out. Mentally ill or not, we all have things that trigger mental deficits.

Another thing that I want to point out is related to high-performing employees that can earn $100,000 or more. It has been proven that they can do this for years at a time because they have built a strong level of resilience. If you're smart, you know that getting or keeping a high-level job takes being resilient in many settings.

People that have high-level jobs are always jumping over hurdles and obstacles, solving problems, and coming to conclusions. The only way to do that is to know your body in and out. If you don't know your triggers in and out, you will never be able to be on the same level as them. Years back, I found out I have to educate and further enlighten myself. If you're doing one thing and it's not working, there comes a point in your life that you have to change your game plan. For me, to get to my eighteenth episode of *Cold Sauce*, I sacrificed a lot. I took time out to build a strong core and learned the fundamentals of this field. I had to find out what made one a good podcaster and a bad podcaster. If you want to be successful, you have to know your field of study in and out.

Some triggers are just a sign of your normal mental health. Some triggers are meant to be prevalent in your life. Some triggers are positive triggers. It takes humbleness to notice the different dimensions of human consciousness. Knowing your triggers can mean testing yourself in different surroundings, how you feel and what draws you on. From my experience, what's triggering you is the thought that's right in front of you. You can't have a mechanism without things that fall apart. There will always be things that throw you off your balance. You have the ability to notice yourself as soon as possible.

PARTIAL OWNERSHIP OF ELEMENTS AROUND YOU

It could be a difficult task for anyone to try to reason with their mentality while reasoning with their consciousness while also trying to be a suitable member of society. It is a task that takes a lot of understanding and experience like knowing who you are, what you need to keep your body up and running, and what implements are needed to function individually. It's very important to understand that there's more to recovery from mental health problems. The simple psychological practices here in this country are giving you a dull-downed form of coping with your problems. Reasoning to cope with living can be a more complex matter. The elements around you and your current form of consciousness form a dynamic duo. They always have an impact on you, whether negative or positive. Most of the successful people in America understand how their body functions and how to reason with their surroundings. They also understand how to correspond with the things around them so they can utilize the tools in a manner that the tools can stay available to them. There are a lot around you that correlates with your mental status. When I first became mentally ill, I had no core understanding of who I was yet. I needed to keep my body functioning properly, my diet correct, and my room clean, especially where to put things so that my consciousness would complement the things around me. For instance, I have a poster right above where I sit. This helps me out greatly because this poster gives me balance. But before I had this poster, I didn't know what parts of the room to place things at. I'm an author and a community spokesman, so I'm always reading, enlightening myself daily and trying to come to a higher form of mentality so I could be a better person for myself and those around me.

You're naturally triggered by different colors also. For instance, I now have colors in my room that complements me. You might not believe this, but all people are triggered by particular colors. Before, I would get negatively affected by certain colors. Also, I have a bulletin board in my room. Before I gained understanding, I didn't know how to properly set up my room. As I told you, I sit and collect my mind and gather thoughts. So what I did was I purchased the bulletin board, and it has alleviated a lot of mental tension in my head. Also, I live in a house with a couple of other family members. My room is upstairs. Before, I also always went downstairs to fix a meal. Over the years, I found out I like things to be close to me. So I bought a portable stovetop in my room, which probably helps me the most. This helped me stay more focused, and I am able to avoid a lot dilemmas this way. This doesn't apply to everybody, but it's important to keep a tight circle. Also, when I was young, books were something I saw no value in. The value of education is priceless. Over the years, I found out that in order for me to be a suitable figure in society, I had to educate myself. So I bought a bookshelf for my room, where I could do cross-referencing. Knowing how to structure your room is probably the most valuable lesson of this episode. I guarantee you that if you structure your room the right way, it's only a matter of time before your mental agony is reduced.

There was a time when I had no core understanding. Knowing how to use the elements around you to your benefit plays a large part in diagnosing your problem. What I haven't spoken on yet is what you input into your mind and what you acquire as valuable data are also like elements around you. How you acquire knowledge and how you shape your mind are very large aspects in diagnosing your mental illness. Your mind is very strong.

A lot of people with a dull-downed state of mind don't know how to acquire knowledge and build themselves mentally. So they view living as something with minimum purpose. You have to strengthen your core value. Coping with mental illness starts with oneself. Once you empower your mind, body, and soul, you then branch off. Then after that branching off, it comes down to how willing you are to stand against the tests of life. What's not mentioned is how your community structure is governed and shaped plays a large part in your consciousness. Every individual is meant to play a part in their community. Their input sheds light on their viewpoints and how they see life. Little things like your street blocks, your stores, the current market in your neighborhood, the availability of your neighborhood, everything about how your neighborhood is structured, you can naturally conceive the properties of the elements in in your setting. A closed mouth doesn't get fed, and neither does an uneducated one. So to make it to the next level of enlightenment, you have to find value in little things. Being well prepared for the role ahead is having prime ownership of your success. Sometimes we forget we live in a fast-paced society in America. It's not all about putting information in your head. It's not *what* you do—it's *how* you do it. Whether you're prepared or not, it's a small iconic suggestibility that grants success. Small things from appliances to setting are all interconnected. A lot of people with mental illness never recover because they never had the stability to fix their problem.

Little things that normal people do can be far out of whack for you. Recovery is generally like a financial investment. What I realized later on is that if I just invested piece by piece, it could have come back to help me. The government is not going to break down the principles, fundamentals, and details about reaching a higher level, which I'm breaking down right now. So I hope you enjoyed and appreciated this podcast. From my experience, how I shaped and valued my room was the largest contribution to my success. A lot of those I grew up with in high school look at me with a little bit of jealousy now because I rose up the ranks and I'm a somebody now. I'm just appreciative that I can express myself and my viewpoints.

THE WEAKNESS OF A STRONG MIND

The name of the game is to educate yourself, empower yourself, and gain the core value of who you are. For those in the mental health community who had their mind shelled once recovered, the test is not over. I wanted to use this episode to say it's not all about putting something in to receive something or being a figure in society that has what it takes to adapt. A very good depiction of this is from the movie *Spider-Man*. In the movie, Spider-Man's uncle Ben tells him, "With great power comes great responsibility." My being able to do all the episodes of *Cold Sauce* is mainly the product of having a large responsibility. It was the study of many kinds. If you want to recover from mental illness one day, put up the best fight possible. The majority of those that are successful in life are in their positions for a reason. Surgeons, doctors, firefighters—these are people that don't have room for error. So the weakness of a strong mind is very important to understand for the mental health community. It's not all about your recovery. From experience, it's about putting up the best fight and then casting that energy on your environment.

In an economy like America's, plenty of people fight for the same resources, and there is so much harshness around that you're looking at a society of people having similar traits. We have to realize that the person that succeeded sacrificed much. If you're part of a community of five thousand, everybody can't hold the same form of employment. You have to sacrifice. At an older age, life forces you to make sacrifices in other ways. In a large sense, to be someone that is heavily fluent in literary studies and has the means to live properly, I have to make several sacrifices. I don't party too much. I sacrificed a large part of my life when I was young to become a community spokesman. In a large sense, I'm very weak in some ways, but very strong in others. I eat right. I make sure I exercise. I don't party too much. I'm not out in public too much. I have to watch my character. I can't live the childlike life that I used to. So just to let you know, there are a lot of sacrifices to having a strong mind.

Another moral of this particular episode is don't be so hard on yourself. It's very important to know every aspect of what keeps your body up and running. For those that emphasize the profit of living, it's only a matter of time, for the most part, before that demeaning mindset deters your body. Oftentimes, being mentally ill means you have a strong mind, but one that hasn't been balanced out yet—a very interesting fact. A good movie that emphasizes this is *A Beautiful Mind*, which is based on a true story. It is about a professor at Princeton University that was so hell-bent on his studies that his mind turned on him. The best way to envision the weakness of a strong mind is to assimilate the powers of a president and envision how his mind is weak in some way. He is somebody that can't slip up character-wise in public. He's strong, but he's also very vulnerable and weak. Like Kanye West mentioned in his song, "The people highest up got the lowest self-esteem." The whole purpose is to empower the mind and body, but to do it in a reasonable fashion.

MONEY ISN'T EVERYTHING

Money is definitely not everything. When you're younger growing up in the communities of America, there is the main fixation of *wanting*. The cost of living right now is at an all-time high. Yes, you do need money. But educated people know the best things in life are free. No one could take the proper standards of living away from you. Some spend too much time worrying about money. The lust for money is why many never recover or seek treatment for their problems. Instead, they seek large sums of money to suit their needs as citizens. It's why many mentally ill patients never see the light or purpose in living. America makes up about 5 percent of the world's population, but also up to 66 percent of the world's psychiatric drugs. You have to understand this is all a scheme. America is perceived as the land of opportunity or the land of great fortune. However, the large number of people hooked on psychiatric drugs should tell you everything you need to know. Money isn't everything, especially when it involves deceiving many people.

A lot of elected officials are deceiving you, making you believe their laws, policies, and acts are credible. You should have some concern over why your neighborhood is counseled the way it is. The value of the dollar is enormous in this country. A lot of Americans don't even realize they've been chasing a carrot on a stick their entire life. Say you are living in the wilderness right now, and you want to have a three-story house, for which you pay about $4,000 a month in mortgage. If you gathered the tools to build that three-story house in the wilderness, you probably could have built the house from the ground up in that setting within a month's time. I understand how money can weaken your mind. For instance, I'm now in a room where I have all the basic necessities I need to run my life. The whole purpose of living is mainly essentials. But in America, you can't see that correlation. Be mindful of this fact: the house or part of the house you're in now you more than likely could have built yourself in a month with materials nearby. Or you could've fed yourself much more easily or had a fair state of living without the need to generate paper currency. Everything sitting in front of me right now that I acquired through money I could have acquired some other way.

Money is nothing with no understanding. For instance, I hear about celebrities and rich people committing suicide all the time. They have large amounts of money stored in the bank. A lot of times, these people don't have the right morals or proper standards of living to withhold that money. A lot of people think that money can make you happy, especially people from low-income neighborhoods. They think money can make them happy. You'd be surprised at how dull-downed the average American mind is. I didn't realize that until I sat still and stopped being so caught up with unrealistic things. There came a point in time when I said, "I need to instill proper lessons in mind to make myself a better person, specifically a better community person." Most mentally ill patients lust for money in the hope that it would help treat their problems. It doesn't. It was said in a documentary about secret societies that most of the elitists that run the world are actually psychopaths. The American chain of command is very narrow. Most of those in US government and others in councils handling world affairs are psychopaths. Take time out to apply your unique regimen and a way to govern yourself to your liking.

YOUNG GRASSHOPPER

I got the meaning behind "young grasshopper" from the '80s movie *The Karate Kid*. I'm sure many of you have seen it or at least heard of it. It is a very inspirational movie. It is about a young boy who was coached by a karate sensei, a martial arts instructor. He was a very spiritual instructor, teaching high forms of discipline and being in tune with your body. He referred to the young boy as "young grasshopper." I found it interesting at that age why he called him that, but I couldn't understand it then. Now I see that calling his young student a "young grasshopper" is very reflective of an everyday citizen's life: the everyday push-and-pull movements and the everyday struggle of navigating life.

I'm sure you've heard of a grasshopper or read about it. A grasshopper has been around since about the Triassic era, about 250 million years ago. Now that I'm older, I caught on to why he referred to this boy as a "young grasshopper." It is a deep idolization of someone with mental problems. A grasshopper is an insect with very precautionary movements. They move in a back-and-forth pace, very determined to get from one point to another. The sensei was referring to a person that moves from one position to the next with much caution. I'm sure many Americans can relate to it. I advise you to pick up the movie *The Karate Kid* yourself. It can teach you a very good lesson on live.

Now that I'm older, I look at my life and the life of others. We are always bent in one direction daily, monthly, or yearly; and all have an opposing force, always dragging you in the opposite direction. If you understand the forces of nature, there will always be a push-and-pull motion.

Not only do I speak on mental concerns that I practice. I also try to bring up an exterior reference that is symbolic and instructive in your place in the world to cope with living. I believe the movements of a grasshopper symbolize a mental state where mental health concerns are not only a predisposition but a normal state of function as well. Being in tune with nature and thinking outside the box are very good things. Through scientific evaluation, it's very hard to be driven at the same speed or at the same levels of force for the majority of your time spent living and not having opposing forces.

Having been around for over 250 million years, grasshoppers certainly are survivors and a species with a unique function. I believe the symbolism of a grasshopper is like a higher form of function, and its relation to a human being also symbolizes taking everything one step at a time and being very careful over the way they live life and use things around them.

If you are of age, sometimes the best way to break out of mental illness is to compare your particular problem to a lively matter around you or a topic of concern. Use that lesson as a way for you to cope with your problems. When I was young, I had serious mental health issues. Now that I'm older, I realize it all had purpose. It's important for someone with mental problems to magnify their problems under a different microscope. That entrenched mindset of mental illness can sometimes be relieved only with in-depth matter that could help you relate to your problems. That's why I chose this particular episode, "Young Grasshopper." Extensive study illustrates the meaning of being precautionary. Each day has to be magnified if you want to make it to the next level of understanding. The instinct and nature of many people around the world are based off being precautionary, which is very similar to those with mental health problems.

VISIT

www.Rootforcepublications.com

<u>The # 1 author website in the U.S.</u>

JOBS. BOOKS. PODCASTS.

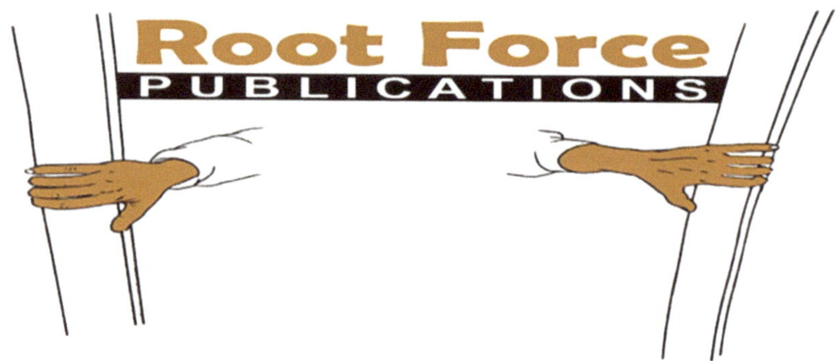

MENTAL HEALTH CONSULTATION.
COMMUNITY OUTREACH. LINKS.

BUY BOOKS WHOLESALE. CONSIGN.
CAREER COACHING.

OR

BUY BOOKS VIA

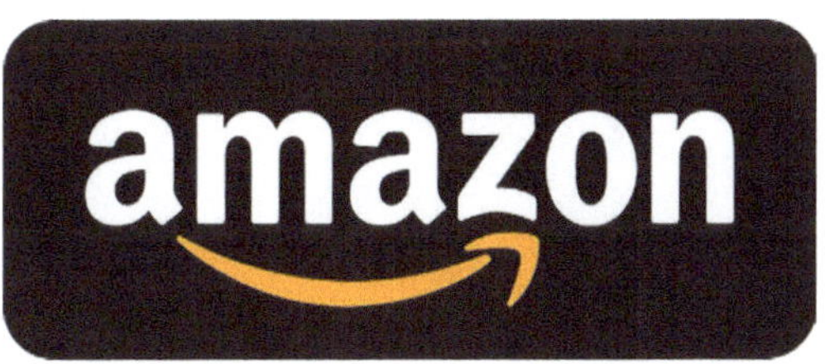

www.Rootforcepublications.com

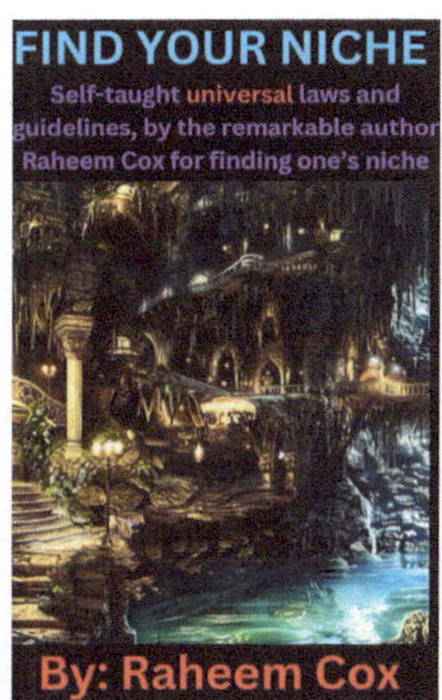

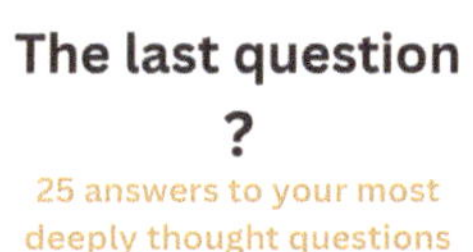

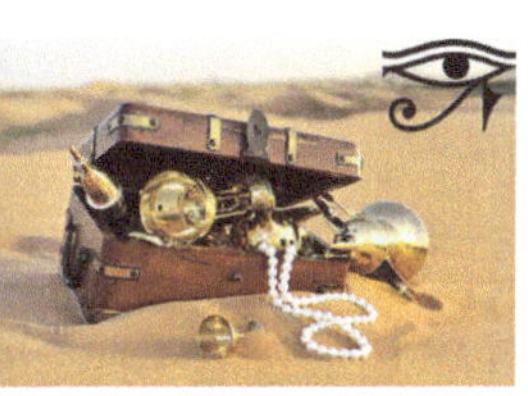

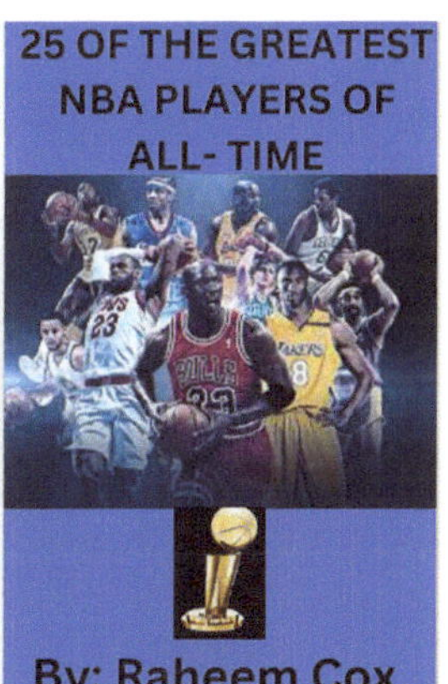

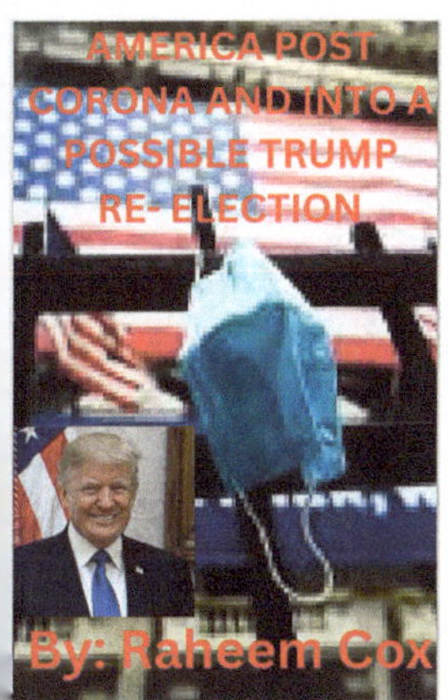

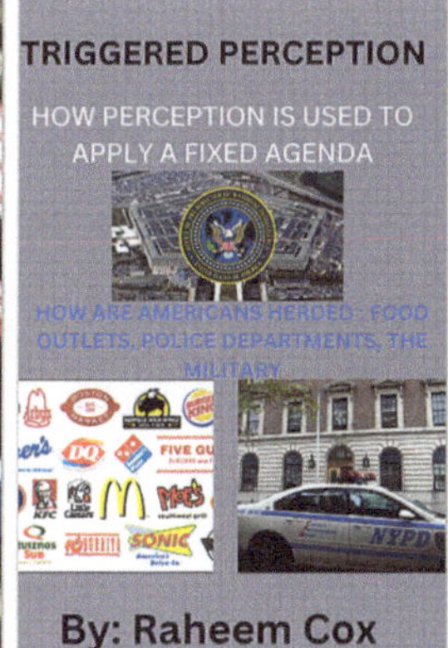

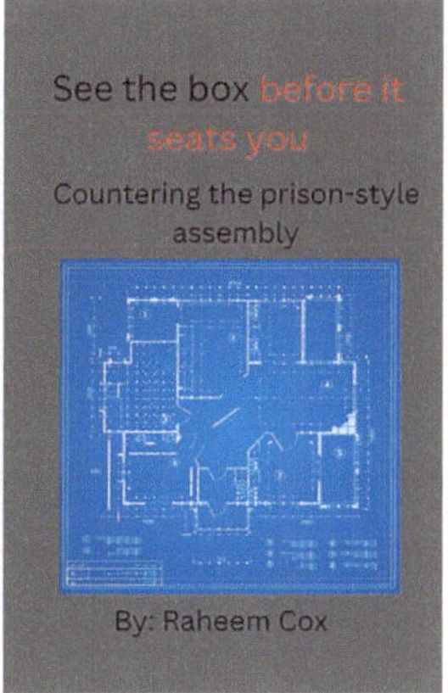

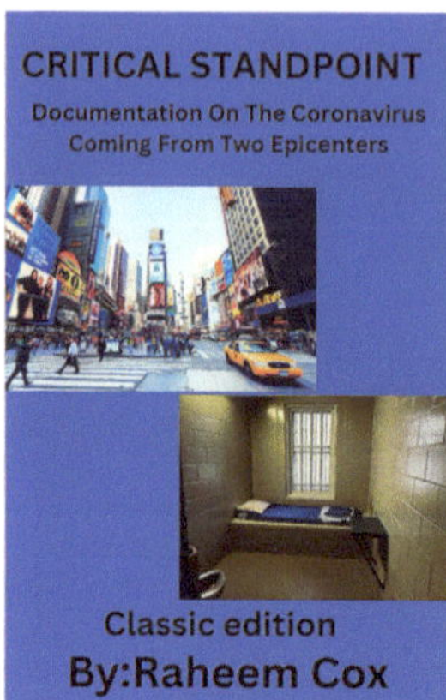

CRITICAL STANDPOINT
Documentation On The Coronavirus Coming From Two Epicenters
Classic edition
By:Raheem Cox

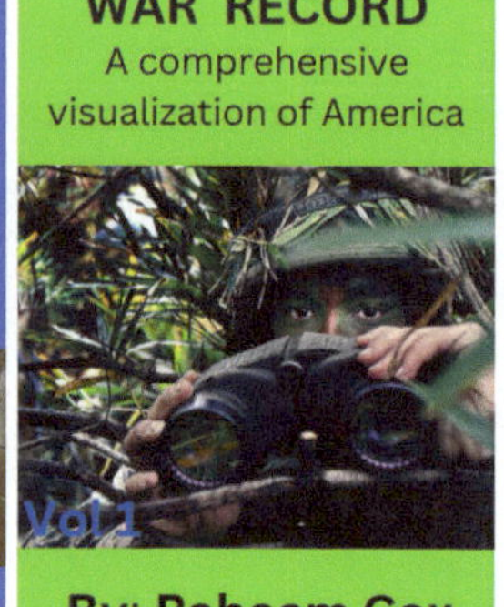

WAR RECORD
A comprehensive visualization of America
Vol 1
By: Raheem Cox

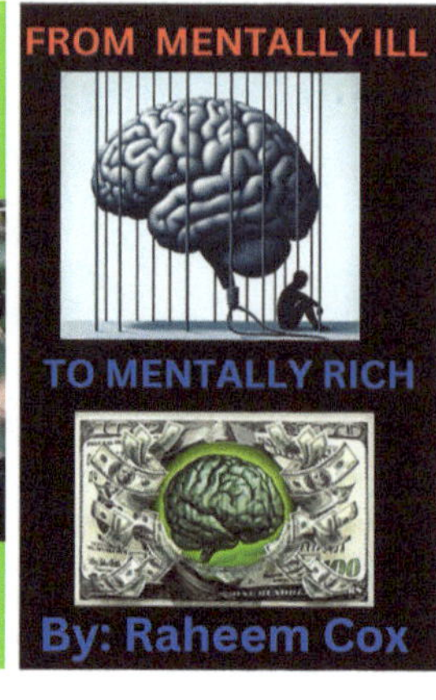

FROM MENTALLY ILL
TO MENTALLY RICH
By: Raheem Cox

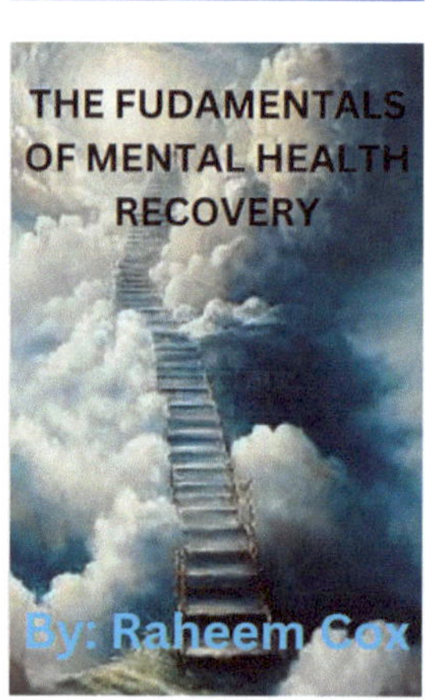

THE FUDAMENTALS OF MENTAL HEALTH RECOVERY
By: Raheem Cox

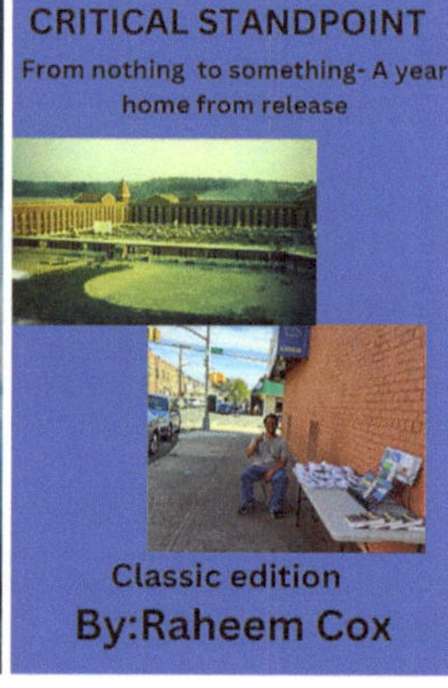

CRITICAL STANDPOINT
From nothing to something- A year home from release
Classic edition
By:Raheem Cox

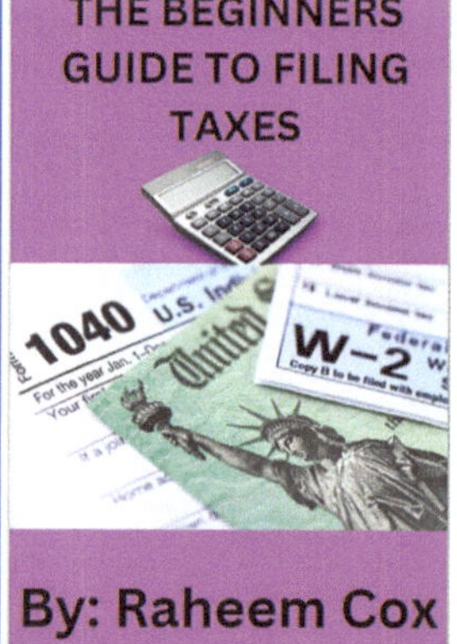

THE BEGINNERS GUIDE TO FILING TAXES
By: Raheem Cox

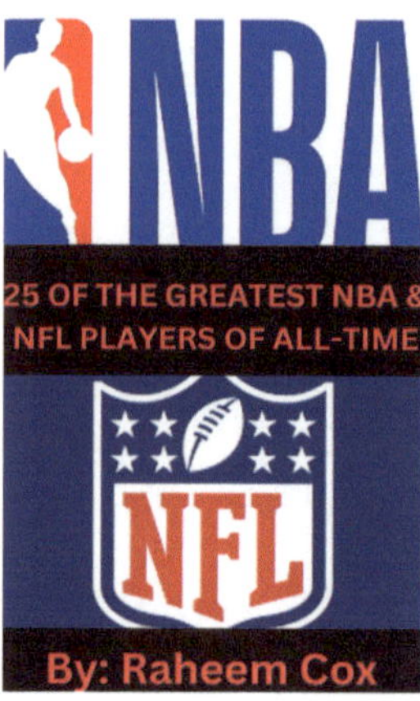

NBA
25 OF THE GREATEST NBA & NFL PLAYERS OF ALL-TIME
NFL
By: Raheem Cox

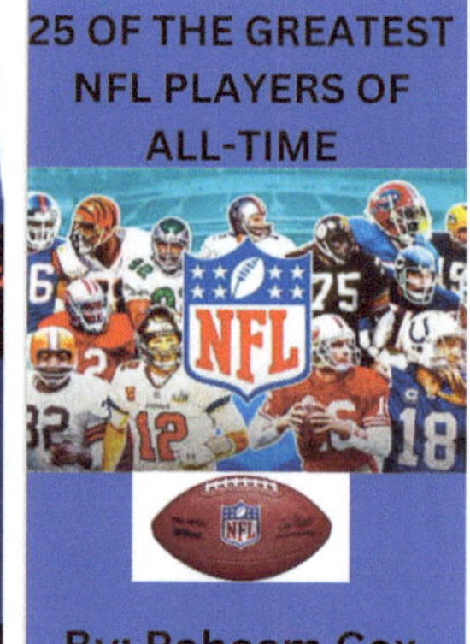

25 OF THE GREATEST NFL PLAYERS OF ALL-TIME
NFL
By: Raheem Cox

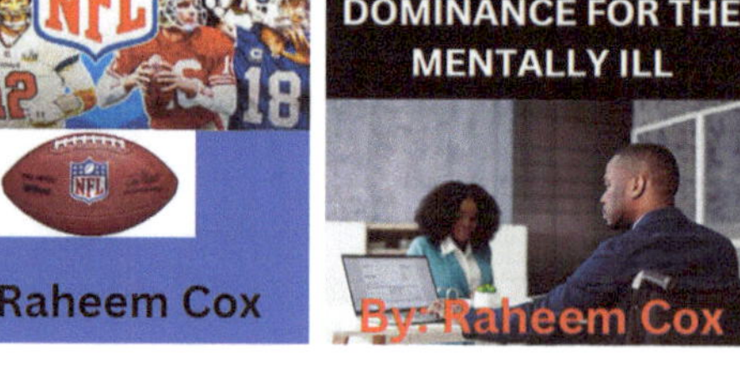

PURSUING MENTAL DOMINANCE FOR THE MENTALLY ILL
By: Raheem Cox